FAST FACTS

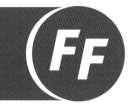

Obstru
Sleep Apnea

Indispensable
Guides to
Clinical
Practice

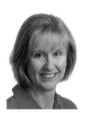

Barbara Phillips MD MSPH
Professor
Division of Pulmonary and Critical Care Medicine
Department of Internal Medicine
University of Kentucky College of Medicine
Lexington, Kentucky, USA

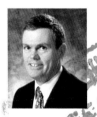

Matthew T Naughton MD FRACP
Associate Professor
Department of Allergy, Immunology and
Respiratory Medicine
Alfred Hospital and Monash University
Melbourne, Victoria, Australia

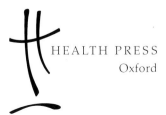

This book is as balanced and as practical as we can make it. Ideas for
improvements are always welcome: feedback@fastfacts.com

HEALTH PRESS
Oxford

Fast Facts – Obstructive Sleep Apnea
First published May 2004

Text © 2004 Barbara Phillips, Matthew T Naughton
© 2004 in this edition Health Press Limited
Health Press Limited, Elizabeth House, Queen Street, Abingdon,
Oxford OX14 3JR, UK
Tel: +44 (0)1235 523233
Fax: +44 (0)1235 523238

Book orders can be placed by telephone or via the website.
For regional distributors or to order via the website, please go to:
www.fastfacts.com
For telephone orders, please call 01752 202301 (UK) or
1 800 538 1287 (North America, toll free).

Fast Facts is a trademark of Health Press Limited.

A CIP catalogue record for this title is available from the British Library.

ISBN 1-903734-47-9

Phillips B (Barbara)
Fast Facts – Obstructive Sleep Apnea/
Barbara Phillips, Matthew T Naughton

Medical illustrations by Dee McLean, London, UK.
Typesetting and page layout by Zed, Oxford, UK.
Printed by Fine Print (Services) Ltd, Oxford, UK.

Printed with vegetable inks on fully biodegradable and
recyclable paper manufactured from sustainable forests.

444   001
Low emissions
during production

Low
chlorine

Sustainable
forests

16145

Glossary of abbreviations

AASM: American Academy of Sleep Medicine (formerly the American Sleep Disorders Association, ASDA)

AHI: apnea–hypopnea index; the total number of episodes of apnea and hypopnea divided by the number of hours of sleep

BiPAP: bilevel positive airway pressure

BMI: body mass index

CAD: coronary artery disease

COPD: chronic obstructive pulmonary disease

CPAP: continuous positive airway pressure

EDS: excessive daytime sleepiness

EEG: electroencephalography

ESS: Epworth Sleepiness Scale

GERD: gastroesophageal reflux disease

NSF: National Sleep Foundation

OSA: obstructive sleep apnea

OSAS: obstructive sleep apnea syndrome

OSAHS: obstructive sleep apnea–hypopnea syndrome

PSG: polysomnography (sleep study)

RDI: Respiratory Disturbance Index, sometimes used interchangeably with AHI

REM: rapid eye movement

RERA: respiratory effort-related arousal

SCN: suprachiasmatic nucleus

SDB: sleep-disordered breathing

SHHS: Sleep Heart Health Study

SL: sleep latency

SSS: Stanford Sleepiness Scale

SWS: slow-wave sleep

UARS: upper airways resistance syndrome

Introduction

The term sleep-disordered breathing (SDB) has been coined to denote the spectrum of respiratory disturbances during sleep, and may include snoring, apneas, hypopneas, increased respiratory effort during sleep, or any combination of sleep-related respiratory disturbances. The terms SDB, sleep apnea, obstructive sleep apnea syndrome (OSAS) and obstructive sleep apnea–hypopnea syndrome are often used interchangeably. We have used the term OSAS throughout.

Obesity and increasing age are significant risk factors for OSAS, but the disorder clearly has both a genetic and a behavioral basis, and there are striking variations in prevalence between ethnic groups. Strong associations have emerged between OSAS and important sequelae, notably automobile accidents and cardiovascular disease. OSAS is also implicated in endocrine derangements, cognitive deficits and mood disorders. Unfortunately, measurement tools for OSAS and definitions of indices of OSAS have not been precise. Recently, however, definitions of OSAS events have been clarified and standardized (see Glossary and Table 4.1, page 41), and the work necessary to validate the terminology and classification is under way.

Several controversies loom with regard to diagnostic tools for OSAS. However, home testing, screening oximetry and clinical algorithms will probably all gain in importance in the future, given the large numbers of patients with OSAS and the growing recognition of the problem. Continuous positive airway pressure (CPAP) remains the treatment of choice, although efforts to address behavioral factors must be part of overall management. Autotitrating CPAP is likely to be at least as effective as CPAP based on laboratory titration. Over time, it is likely that the diagnosis and treatment of OSAS will become more streamlined and empirical, since the disorder is common and deadly, but treatment is effective, safe and inexpensive.

Breathing during sleep constitutes a spectrum with no clear boundaries between pathological and normal (Figure 1.1). The mildest form of SDB is intermittent snoring, which may be a nuisance without significant health consequences; however, evidence that chronic snoring may have significant effects is accumulating. At the other end of the spectrum, the most severe form of SDB is the obesity–hypoventilation syndrome (formerly called Pickwickian syndrome), which is associated with severe morbidity and very high mortality. Between these two extremes are disorders with gradually increasing impact on morbidity and mortality: persistent snoring, upper airway resistance syndrome and OSAS.

Prevalence

Both the prevalence and awareness of breathing disturbances during sleep have increased markedly in recent years, partly owing to significant advances in diagnosis and treatment. However, two developments over the last decade have undoubtedly contributed: the increase in the prevalence of obesity and the age of the

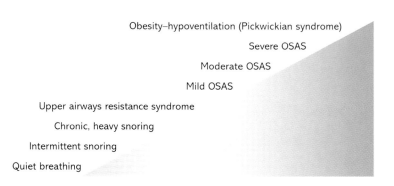

Obesity–hypoventilation (Pickwickian syndrome)

Severe OSAS

Moderate OSAS

Mild OSAS

Upper airways resistance syndrome

Chronic, heavy snoring

Intermittent snoring

Quiet breathing

Figure 1.1 The spectrum of breathing during sleep. OSAS, obstructive sleep apnea syndrome.

population. The best current estimate of the prevalence of clinically significant OSAS in developed countries is about 5%.

The classic Wisconsin Sleep Cohort Study of 3513 subjects, aged 30–60 years, found that 44% of men and 28% of women were habitual snorers (Table 1.1). In this cohort, 4% of men and 2% of women had OSAS, defined as an apnea–hypopnea index (AHI) of greater than 5, associated with daytime hypersomnolence.

In the landmark Sleep Heart Health Study (SHHS), the median AHI was 4.4. Since an AHI of 5 or more is often used as the cutoff for significant OSAS, nearly half of the SHHS cohort of over 6000 individuals in their early 60s met the criteria for OSAS!

Risk factors

Obesity is the most important risk factor for OSAS in Caucasians, and the risk of significant OSAS rises with body mass index (BMI). About 40% of those with a BMI of 40 and 50% of those with a BMI of 50 have significant OSAS.

It is likely that obesity is a more important risk factor for OSAS in middle-aged women than it is in men, whereas age may be a more important risk factor for men. Simply put, a premenopausal woman with OSAS is generally more obese than her male counterpart.

TABLE 1.1

Results of the Wisconsin Sleep Cohort Study of middle-aged subjects (30–60 years)

	Prevalence (%)	
	Men	Women
Self-reported excessive daytime sleepiness	16	23
Habitual snoring	44	28
AHI > 5	24	9
AHI > 5 plus excessive daytime sleepiness	4	2

AHI, apnea–hypopnea index (total number of episodes of apnea and hypopnea divided by the number of hours of sleep).

Age. The prevalence of OSAS increases with increasing age (Figure 1.2). Early studies found that the prevalence of sleep apnea in the elderly was 24–73%. While studies of clinical populations have tended to find a peak prevalence of clinically significant OSAS in middle age, population-based studies have found increasing levels of OSAS with aging, even though obesity is less prevalent with increasing age.

Before the age of about 50, men are roughly twice as likely as women to have OSAS. This gap in the prevalence of OSAS decreases after the menopause, because women appear to have a greater age-related risk and thus an increase in the prevalence of apnea after the menopause. After the menopause, both gender and age become much less important risk factors.

Family history. Studies have shown a much higher prevalence of OSAS among offspring of family members with OSAS, compared with the general population. A large twin study has confirmed that there is a substantial genetic contribution to self-reported snoring

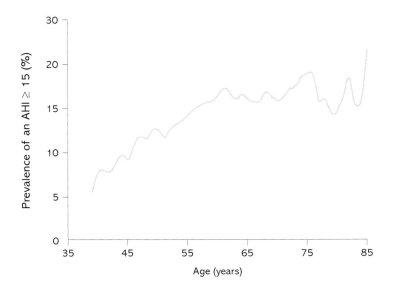

Figure 1.2 The prevalence of OSAS increases with increasing age. Data from Young et al. 2002. AHI, apnea–hypopnea index.

and sleepiness in older men, even when controlling for obesity. Furthermore, the Human Genome Project has established a genetic predisposition to OSAS and identified several specific loci. However, as with many heritable tendencies, most individuals who carry the implicated gene(s) are not afflicted with the condition. Environmental factors apparently 'turn on' genes to cause expression of disease.

Race. OSAS appears to be more prevalent in certain races. Several investigators have identified an increased prevalence of OSAS in African-Americans of all ages. OSAS also appears to be more prevalent in Asian and Hispanic individuals. These ethnic variations in the risk of OSAS persist even when results are controlled for other risk factors, notably BMI.

Hormones. Hypothyroidism is more prevalent in individuals with OSAS, and may contribute to the development of OSAS by several mechanisms, including obesity, increased tongue size and reduced respiratory drive. Between 1.4 and 4% of those diagnosed with OSAS have previously unsuspected hypothyroidism.

Airway caliber. Although the evidence is not overwhelming, nasal obstruction and rhinitis are also associated with increased snoring and OSAS. OSAS should be strongly suspected in the craniofacial syndromes that affect airway caliber such as acromegaly, trisomy 21 (Down's syndrome), Pierre Robin, Alpert's, Treacher Collins and Marfan's syndromes.

Neck size. Recent attention has focused on the increased prevalence of snoring, sleepiness and OSAS in professional American football players. Although these individuals tend to have large BMIs (and to be male), they are generally fit. They do, however, have increased neck sizes as a result of deliberate training (and possibly anabolic steroid use) to increase neck strength. Neck circumference is highly predictive of the risk of OSAS (see page 18), and the data from football players suggests that increased neck circumference plays a key role in the development of OSAS.

Behavioral factors are also risk factors for the development and increased severity of OSAS. Alcohol and sedative medications (including most hypnotics) decrease upper airway neuromuscular drive, predisposing to recurrent upper airway collapse. Even modest alcohol consumption significantly increases both the heart rate and the frequency of OSA during sleep. Tobacco smoke causes an increase in nasal and pharyngeal irritation, resulting in edema and narrowing of the upper airway. It also increases mucus production, which contributes to upper airway obstruction. Furthermore, cigarette smoking causes alveolar destruction and ventilation–perfusion mismatching, which can increase the severity of oxygen desaturation associated with reduced or absent airflow during sleep.

Key points – epidemiology and risk factors

- The prevalence of sleep apnea is about 5% and increasing.
- Obesity is the most important risk factor for sleep apnea.
- Cigarette smoking and drinking alcohol increase the risk and severity of OSAS.
- There is a genetic predisposition to OSAS.

Key references

Li KK, Powell NB, Kushida C et al. A comparison of Asian and white patients with obstructive sleep apnea syndrome. *Laryngoscope* 1999;109: 1937–40.

Palmer LJ, Buxbaum SG, Larkin E et al. A whole-genome scan for obstructive sleep apnea and obesity. *Am J Hum Genet* 2003;72:340–50

Shahar E, Redline S, Young T et al. for the Sleep Heart Health Study. Hormone replacement therapy and sleep-disordered breathing. *Am J Crit Care Med* 2003;167:1186–92.

Shahar E, Whitney CW, Redline S et al. Sleep-disordered breathing and cardiovascular disease. Cross-sectional results of the Sleep Heart Health Study. *Am J Respir Crit Care Med* 2001;163:19–25.

Tischler PV, Larkin EK, Schluchter MD, Redline S. Incidence of sleep-disordered breathing in an urban adult population. The relative importance of risk factors in the development of sleep-disordered breathing. *JAMA* 2003;289:2230–7.

Wetter DW, Young TB, Bidwell TR et al. Smoking as a risk factor for sleep-disordered breathing. *Arch Intern Med* 1994;154:2219–24.

Young T, Shahar E, Nieto FJ et al. Sleep Heart Health Study Research Group. Predictors of sleep-disordered breathing in community-dwelling adults: the Sleep Heart Health Study. *Arch Intern Med* 2002:22;162:893–900.

Young T, Peppard PE, Gottlieb DJ. Epidemiology of obstructive sleep apnea. *Am J Respir Crit Care Med* 2002;165:1217–39.

The spectrum of SDB varies from simple intermittent snoring to obnoxiously severe snoring associated with OSAS and cardiovascular sequelae, through to orthopnea, paroxysmal nocturnal dyspnea and fragmented sleep associated with unstable or decompensated cardiovascular and/or pulmonary disease. This chapter will concentrate on the snoring and OSAS end of this spectrum. Central sleep apnea (most commonly presenting as Cheyne–Stokes respiration) will not be discussed in detail here, but is reviewed in the section on congestive heart failure (page 25).

OSAS is a common disorder that can present in varied ways, but is generally recognized when:
- others complain of the snoring noise
- medical complications of apnea arise
- cognitive performance decreases or sleepiness sufficient to impair performance develops (most commonly noticed when it causes an accident).

The clinical consequences of OSAS result from sleep disturbance and/or hypoxemia.

History

Heavy snoring is the most common symptom in patients with OSAS. However, about half of men and a quarter of women snore, but somewhat fewer than that have OSAS, so snoring alone is not diagnostic. Snoring accompanied by apnea, snorting, gasping and choking during sleep is predictive of OSAS (Table 2.1). Witnessed apneas are more predictive of OSAS than are self-reported episodes of waking up gasping for breath, which may be a symptom of other diseases, such as congestive heart failure, gastroesophageal reflux disease, nocturnal asthma or panic disorder.

Snoring. Most snorers are unaware that they are a problem to others or to themselves until they share a sleeping space with

TABLE 2.1

Symptoms and signs of obstructive sleep apnea syndrome

Symptoms

- Snoring
- Witnessed apneas
- Gasping for breath during sleep
- Sleepiness
- Enuresis, nocturia
- Mood, memory or learning problems
- Erectile dysfunction
- Recent weight gain
- Morning headache
- Dry mouth or throat in the morning

Signs

- Obesity
- Hypertension
- Crowded oropharynx
- Retrognathia

someone else (Figure 2.1). The snoring sound may exceed 85 decibels, which is similar to the sound of a busy road, and may disturb people even one or two rooms away. Periods of silence may reflect either the resumption of normal breathing or pathological apneas. The intensity and tone of snoring varies depending on the site of airway collapse and the strength of the inspiratory muscles.

The earliest age that snoring can occur parallels the development of speech (about 18 months), when the upper airway becomes increasingly flexible as a result of the separation of the soft palate from the epiglottis. In children with a normal craniofacial structure, the peak incidence of snoring is 3–6 years, which corresponds to an age when the ratio of upper airway lymphoid tissue to craniofacial size is greatest.

(a)

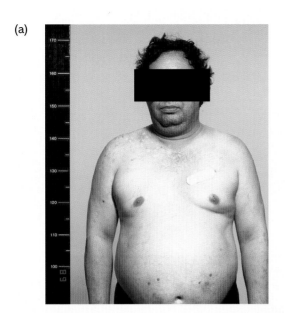

(b)

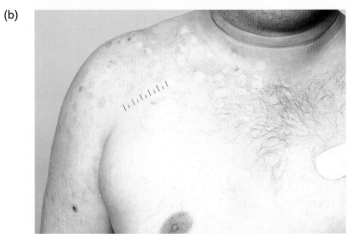

Figure 2.1 (a) A 40-year-old obese male who presented with acute myocardial infarction. During the period of monitoring, his loud snoring would disrupt staff and other patients. He was diagnosed with severe obstructive sleep apnea syndrome and treated successfully with continuous positive airway pressure.
(b) The hypopigmented lesions on the patient's right upper chest wall and arm are burns caused by cigarettes dropping from his mouth when he fell asleep.

15

The elderly are also predisposed to snoring and OSAS as a result of weight gain, side effects of medication (e.g. sedatives, analgesics, muscle relaxants), loss of muscle tone or the development of associated medical problems that might exacerbate the apnea (e.g. hypothyroidism). However, age-related loss of muscle strength reduces the overall inspiratory pressure (required to generate loud snoring sounds) and thus diminishes the loudness of snoring.

Snoring can, therefore, occur at any time from childhood to old age. It is also likely that the longer one snores, the greater the risk of developing cardiovascular disease or having accidents related to sleep fragmentation (Figure 2.1). Thus, someone who begins to snore in childhood with fragmented sleep is more likely to develop the medical complications of OSAS.

Snoring should be taken seriously if it occurs more frequently than two nights/week, is loud enough to be audible in other rooms or to make a bed partner move to a separate room, or is associated with witnessed apneas, dyspnea or choking (Table 2.2). Snoring that occurs in lateral as well as supine sleeping positions or that is associated with medical disorders or neurocognitive impairment is also of concern.

Sleepiness

Excessive daytime sleepiness should increase suspicion of OSAS. Subjective sleepiness may be assessed using the Epworth Sleepiness

TABLE 2.2

When snoring may have serious consequences

- It is audible in another room
- It occurs more than two nights/week
- It occurs when the person is lying in a lateral position
- It is associated with apneas
- It is associated with cardiovascular disease
- It is associated with excessive daytime sleepiness
- It is associated with structural upper airway pathology

Scale (ESS; Table 2.3), which has been validated in clinical studies and correlates with objective measures of sleepiness. An ESS score greater than 10 suggests significant daytime sleepiness, but is not specific for OSAS. Patients both under- and over-report their own sleepiness, so questioning partners or family may also be useful.

Sleepiness can also be objectively measured by the Multiple Sleep Latency Test, but this is seldom indicated in the evaluation of OSAS.

TABLE 2.3

The Epworth Sleepiness Scale

How likely are you to doze off or fall asleep in the following situations, in contrast to just feeling tired? This refers to your usual way of life in recent times. Even if you have not done some of these things recently, try to work out how they would have affected you.

Use the following scale to choose the most appropriate number for each situation:

0 = would *never* doze; 1 = *slight* chance of dozing; 2 = *moderate* chance of dozing; 3 = *high* chance of dozing.

Situation	Chance of dozing
Sitting and reading	_____
Watching TV	_____
Sitting, inactive, in a public place	_____
As a passenger in a car for an hour	_____
Lying down in the afternoon	_____
Sitting and talking to someone	_____
Sitting quietly after a lunch without alcohol	_____
In a car, while stopped for a few minutes in traffic	_____

Patients who report falling asleep while driving should be evaluated for sleep disorders including OSAS. Many sleep problems, including chronic, self-imposed sleep deprivation, may result in falling asleep while driving. As this symptom poses a threat both to the patient and others, clinicians should have a low threshold for evaluation of patients who report falling asleep while driving.

Nocturia, erectile dysfunction, attention deficits, cognitive impairment (see below) and morning headache or dry or sore throat are other symptoms that may be associated to varying degrees with the presence of OSAS. Recent weight gain is an almost invariable finding, and may be both the cause and the consequence of OSAS.

Physical findings

Obesity. The physical finding that is most predictive of OSAS is central obesity (Figure 2.1). A BMI of 28 in both men and women should increase suspicion of OSAS. Roughly 40% of individuals with a BMI over 40 and 50% of those with a BMI over 50 have significant OSAS, though premenopausal female patients are generally much heavier than their male counterparts, and both obesity and gender become less important risk factors for OSAS after 50 years of age.

Neck size. Measures of central obesity, such as neck size, are very useful in predicting the presence of OSAS. In men with a neck size of 43 cm (17") or greater and women with a neck size of 40 cm (16") or greater, OSAS is very likely to be confirmed by overnight polysomnography.

Nasal obstruction from any cause appears to be a risk for OSAS, including snoring. A narrowed posterior oropharynx, deviated septum, retrognathia and other craniofacial abnormalities that result in airway narrowing are frequently seen in patients with OSAS. Craniofacial abnormalities may range from subtle (e.g. mild retrognathia, narrow maxilla) to severe in a number of syndromes (Table 2.4).

Importantly, OSAS may occur in a non-obese patient (Figure 2.2). Several diagnostic schemes are based on intra-oral

TABLE 2.4

Craniofacial abnormalities predisposing to sleep apnea

- Retrognathia/micrognathia
- Maxillary insufficiency
- Marfan's syndrome
- Narrow face and high arched palate
- Pierre Robin syndrome
- Treacher Collins syndrome
- Alpert's syndrome
- Hurler's syndrome
- Hunter's syndrome
- Cerebral palsy
- Trisomy 21 (Down's syndrome)
- Prader–Willi syndrome

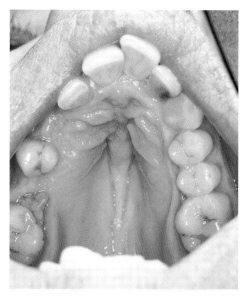

Figure 2.2 Obstructive sleep apnea syndrome can occur in a non-obese patient with a high arched palate that places the tongue posteriorly and inferiorly, and encroaches on the nasal space.

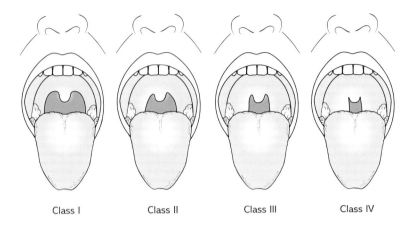

| Class I | Class II | Class III | Class IV |

Figure 2.3 A pharyngeal grading system for assessing the physical findings of airway narrowing in obstructive sleep apnea syndrome. Reproduced with permission from Tsai et al. 2003.

measurements that basically show a narrowed airway in the posterior oropharynx (Figure 2.3).

Hypertension. Recent large epidemiological studies that have controlled for important confounders, including obesity, have

---

Key points – clinical presentation

- Snoring is a common but non-specific symptom of sleep-disordered breathing.
- Sleepiness is common in patients with obstructive sleep apnea syndrome, but has many other causes.
- A history of witnessed apneas is a robust predictor of the likelihood of obstructive sleep apnea syndrome.
- Neck circumference (> 43 cm [17"] in a man or > 40 cm [16"] in a woman) predicts an increased likelihood of sleep apnea.
- The prevalence of hypertension is greater in patients with obstructive sleep apnea syndrome than in the general population.

clearly demonstrated that OSAS is a risk factor for hypertension in a 'dose-dependent' manner (see Chapter 3).

Key references

Davies RJ, Ali NJ, Stradling JR. Neck circumference and other clinical features in the diagnosis of the obstructive sleep apnoea syndrome. *Thorax* 1992;47: 101–5.

Johns MW. A new method for measuring daytime sleepiness: the Epworth sleepiness scale. *Sleep* 1991;14:540–5.

Peppard PE, Young T, Palta M, Skatrud J. Prospective study of the association between sleep-disordered breathing and hypertension. *N Engl J Med* 2000;342:1378–84.

Rowley JA, Aboussouan LS, Badr S. The use of clinical prediction formulae in the evaluation of obstructive sleep apnea. *Sleep* 2000;23:929–38.

Tsai WH, Remmers JE, Brant R et al. A decision rule for diagnostic testing in obstructive sleep apnea. *Am J Respir Crit Care Med* 2003;167:1427–32.

The most prominent medical complications of OSAS cited in the current medical literature are cardiovascular. Even when age, gender, obesity, and cigarette and alcohol consumption are controlled for, OSAS is associated with systemic hypertension, coronary artery disease (CAD) and cerebrovascular disease. Importantly, the healthcare costs of untreated OSAS patients are much greater than those of patients without OSAS, and decline significantly to non-OSAS levels once OSAS treatment has been instigated.

Systemic hypertension

The association between systemic hypertension and OSAS has been known for decades. Recently, the cause-and-effect relationship has been confirmed, and is independent of age, BMI, gender, alcohol consumption and cigarette use. Compared with healthy control subjects without OSAS, the odds ratios of OSAS patients developing systemic hypertension over a 4-year period are 1.42, 2.03 and 2.89 for AHIs of 0–5, 5–15 and > 15 at baseline, respectively. The prevalence of OSAS is particularly high in patients with drug-resistant hypertension; in one study, OSAS was diagnosed in 83% of patients who had uncontrolled hypertension despite taking three or more antihypertensive agents. Furthermore, treatment of OSAS with CPAP is associated with a fall in mean systemic blood pressure of 10 mmHg. Thus, OSAS is now recognized as a cause of hypertension.

Epidemiological studies suggest that approximately 40% of patients with systemic hypertension have OSAS; similarly, about 40% of OSAS patients have systemic hypertension. The approximations are partly due to the varied definitions of both OSAS and systemic hypertension. There is considerable interlaboratory variation in the definitions and thresholds used for sleep apnea (see Chapter 4). Similarly, problems in identifying hypertension can occur because:

- blood pressure is usually measured while the patient is awake, yet the first sign of hypertension is the loss of the approximately 20 mmHg nocturnal dip in blood pressure
- ambulatory blood pressure devices, which inflate a cuff every 15–60 minutes over a 24-hour period, wake patients from sleep with each cuff inflation.

Furthermore, data on hypertension are usually based on questionnaires – 'Do you have high blood pressure?', 'Do you attend regular medical check-ups for hypertension?' and 'Do you take medication for hypertension?' – which patients may not understand well enough to answer reliably.

Despite these limitations, there is compelling evidence that OSAS is a cause of systemic hypertension. Several mechanisms have been proposed.

- Hypoxia and hypercapnia induce elevation of sympathetic nervous system activity, initially during sleep, and later during wakefulness.
- Loss or resetting of baroreceptor activity occurs as a result of recurrent large negative intrathoracic pressure swings during apnea. Loss of baroreceptor (vagal) activity means that sympathetic tone is unopposed.
- Recurrent surges in sympathetic activity associated with apnea terminating in arousal are also associated with acute elevations in blood pressure.
- Endothelial damage results from hypoxia and possibly hyperoxia, which reduces the production and release of some of the naturally occurring vasodilators, such as nitric oxide.
- Fluid and salt imbalance associated with the kidneys, caused by alterations in the renin–angiotensin system and atrial natriuretic peptide levels, can promote elevated blood pressure.

Identification of OSAS and treatment with CPAP have resulted in significant falls in mean 24-hour blood pressure (measured via inflated cuff or continuously with finger photoplethysmography) of between 3 and 10 mmHg within 4–8 weeks. Importantly, such falls translate into a reduction in the lifetime risk of future cardiovascular events of more than 30%.

Coronary artery disease

Both OSAS and CAD are common disorders. In middle-aged populations (30–60 years), OSAS and CAD occur in 24% and 20% of men, and 9% and 6% of women, respectively. Risk factors common to both conditions are male gender, obesity, increasing age, cigarette smoking and diabetes mellitus.

The lifetime risk of myocardial infarction in patients with OSAS, independent of age, BMI and blood pressure, is increased fivefold according to recent studies. Moreover, the chance of surviving a myocardial infarct is worse for patients with OSAS than for non-OSAS patients. In one study, 75% of patients with angiographically proven CAD had OSAS. Importantly, treatment with CPAP reduces the symptoms of CAD, particularly those related to nocturnal angina.

Patients with little or no CAD may exhibit ST changes during sleep (Figure 3.1). Whether this is due to OSAS and impaired oxygen delivery or to exacerbation of a subtle (< 50%), preexisting narrowing of a coronary artery remains to be determined. Other causes of ST changes apart from myocardial ischemia, such as electrolyte disorders, increased sympathetic nervous system activity and changes in body position, should be considered.

Whether OSAS contributes to the pathogenesis of CAD is unclear, but several mechanisms, listed here, have been proposed.

- The direct effects of hypoxemia on the endothelial wall promote and accelerate atherosclerosis.
- The indirect effects of reduced oxygen delivery to the myocardium starve it of oxygen.
- Impaired myocardial perfusion is the result of tachycardia and reduced diastole.
- Large, negative intrathoracic pressures related to apnea increase the left ventricular wall pressure gradient, thus reducing myocardial perfusion. Similarly, at the time of arousal, systemic vasoconstriction occurs with a resultant rise in blood pressure.

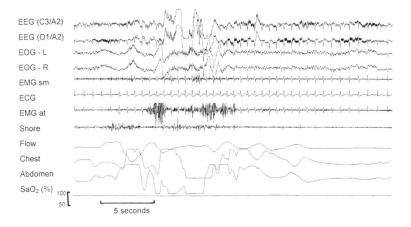

Figure 3.1 A 30-second display from a polysomnogram of a patient with angina. Note the ST depression that occurs with the arousal that terminates a hypopnea.

Both negative intrathoracic pressures and peripheral vasoconstriction lead to increased left ventricular afterload, and thus increased myocardial work and greater oxygen demands.

- The large negative intrathoracic pressures during an episode of apnea are associated with cardiac chamber distortion. The coronary vessels that overlie the myocardium are also exposed to distorting pressures, which could lead to plaque rupture.
- Elevated sympathetic activity and OSAS are both associated with increased blood coagulability, which could precipitate coronary artery occlusion (plaque rupture and clot formation) in the setting of increased demand, but reduced availability, of oxygen.

Congestive heart failure

The cardinal feature of congestive heart failure (CHF) is dyspnea that occurs on exercise, at rest or asleep in the supine position and, in severe cases, while awake and upright. The mechanism by which dyspnea occurs during sleep is largely due to either OSA (Figure 3.2) or central sleep apnea (CSA).

Unlike OSA, CSA is not caused by an obstruction, but by a disorder of the central drive to ventilation, which results from a 'circulatory delay' and an exaggerated ventilatory response to chemical stimuli (e.g. carbon dioxide) during stages 1 and 2 non-rapid-eye-movement (non-REM) sleep, when respiratory control is

(a)

(b)

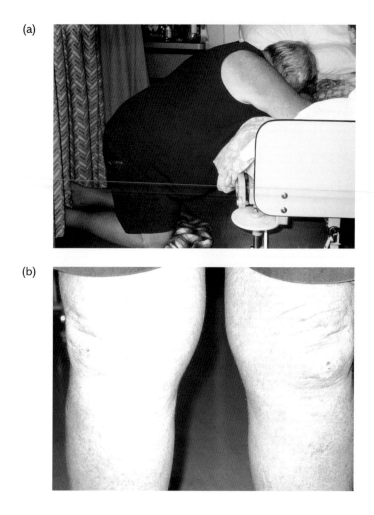

Figure 3.2 A 55-year-old long-haul truck driver had been diagnosed and treated for heart failure for 3 years. He had slept kneeling by his bed for at least 5 years, because he said his neck closed over when he lay in bed. As a consequence, his kneecaps had ulcerated. He was diagnosed with severe obstructive sleep apnea syndrome and treated successfully with continuous positive airway pressure.

under chemical control. A delay in oxygenated arterial blood leaving the pulmonary circulation and being detected by the peripheral and central chemosensors (carotid body and medulla, respectively) is due to an enlarged left ventricle and atrium, and reduced contraction during systole. A prolongation of the circulation time from 10 seconds to more than 20 seconds can result in a 180° phase shift in the control of ventilation. An exaggerated ventilatory response to carbon dioxide will allow the prevailing partial pressure of carbon dioxide in arterial blood (Pa_{CO_2}) to fall transiently below the apnea threshold and thus result in a temporary cessation of ventilation until the Pa_{CO_2} levels rise and hyperventilation resumes. The cyclic central apnea–hyperpnea results in a typical waxing and waning pattern of ventilation during non-REM sleep called Cheyne–Stokes respiration.

Patients with CHF commonly exhibit both OSA and CSA, but each form of apnea has characteristic features. CSA is associated with less obesity, greater atrial fibrillation, greater male predominance, a lower Pa_{CO_2} both when awake and asleep, and higher pulmonary capillary wedge pressure and sympathetic nervous system activity (e.g. circulating catecholamines). Thus, CSA is thought to be associated with more severe CHF and possibly increased mortality. CSA patients commonly present with orthopnea or paroxysmal nocturnal dyspnea with witnessed apneas, and often complain of insomnia and anxiety. Frequently, snoring is absent. In contrast, OSAS patients fit the more commonly observed morphology of the snoring, obese male.

It is important to differentiate CSA from OSAS for the following clinical reasons.

- Aggressive medical therapy (including correction of bradycardic conditions with a pacemaker or heart transplant) can attenuate CSA severity.
- CSA and OSAS commonly coexist; removal or treatment of CSA may unmask moderate-to-severe OSAS. In some CHF patients, the apnea may change from OSA to CSA within the same night, presumably because of a gradual deterioration in heart function as the night progresses.

- CSA and OSA respond differently to CPAP. OSA ceases immediately, whereas CSA responds over days to weeks in response to the improvement in cardiac function associated with CPAP.

Cerebrovascular disease

Sleep apnea is more common in patients who have had a stroke and/or transient ischemic attacks than in the general population. In these patients, the apnea is predominantly obstructive rather than central. The prevalence of OSAS is about 75% in the first few weeks after a stroke and decreases to about 35% at 3 months. It is unclear why the prevalence diminishes, but it may be explained by correction of some apnea-aggravating factors, such as supine body position, alcohol consumption, excess weight and sedative use. Alternatively, it may be related to the resolution of stroke and improved neural control of ventilation.

The prevalence of OSAS appears to be independent of stroke site and type (i.e. ischemic or hemorrhagic). CSA, however, is seen in the approximately 15% of stroke patients with coexisting cardiac disease (CHF or atrial fibrillation).

As OSAS causes systemic hypertension, and hypertension is one of the leading causes of stroke, it is likely that OSAS contributes to the etiology of stroke in this way. Other mechanisms may include: vibration of the carotid arteries (patients with OSAS are more likely to have calcified carotid arteries than non-snorers); increased platelet aggregation related to sympathetic activity; transient atrial fibrillation during sleep; and altered cerebral autoregulation due to changes in arterial blood gas levels.

Nerve damage

Some patients with OSAS may have symptoms of upper airway discomfort, and some patients are known to have local upper airway sensory neuropathy. Detailed nerve testing has also demonstrated peripheral sensory neuropathy in patients with OSAS and, therefore, recurrent systemic hypoxia followed by hyperoxia and oxygen radical formation are thought to cause nerve damage.

The upper airway may also become neuropathic as a result of local trauma from snoring.

Cardiac arrhythmias

A number of cardiac arrhythmias are seen in patients with OSAS (Table 3.1).

Considerable heart rate variability is commonly seen during sleep monitoring, with bradycardia during episodes of OSA (diving reflex) and tachycardia during arousals. Periods of sinus pause of up to 2.5 seconds are often reported. In the absence of periodic limb movements, patterns of heart rate variability can be used diagnostically to differentiate normal ventilation during sleep from sleep apnea, and possibly to differentiate CSA from OSA. Younger, healthy adults with intact baroreceptors will demonstrate considerable heart rate variability, often in the absence of hypoxemia. In older patients, however, baroreceptor activity may have been attenuated after years of untreated OSAS, leading to a loss of heart rate variability and prominent hypoxemia with each respiratory event.

In a recent study, 18% of patients with OSAS (randomly selected irrespective of cardiac history) had cardiac arrhythmias. These included brief sinus pauses, extraventricular beats (salvos of 3 or more and bigeminy), as well as second- and third-degree heart

TABLE 3.1

Cardiac arrhythmias observed in patients with obstructive sleep apnea syndrome

- Loss of heart rate variability
- Sinus arrhythmia
- Sinus pause < 2.5 seconds
- Ventricular extrasystoles (salvos, bigeminy, unifocal and multifocal)
- Atrial tachycardias (transient atrial fibrillation, atrial extrasystoles)
- Heart block (first, second and third degree)
- Sinus arrest (usually < 13 seconds)

block. Notably, these arrhythmias occurred only at nighttime and were reversed in all patients (except one who had an incidental finding of aortic stenosis) by the application of nasal CPAP.

Less commonly, periods of sinus pause of up to 13 seconds have been reported during the apneic episode. In such patients, OSAS and additional factors (e.g. medication, conduction defect, hypothyroidism) may be contributory.

Tachyarrhythmias are seen in about 1–5 % of OSAS patients and include transient atrial fibrillation and periodic and self-limiting ventricular tachycardia. Recently, in a group of patients with recent onset atrial fibrillation and known OSAS, the rate of recurrence of the atrial fibrillation was halved when the OSAS was effectively treated. Frequent, premature atrial and ventricular ectopic beats commonly occur in patients with OSAS, but are of dubious clinical significance. However, the mean heart rate during sleep provides important information about autonomic control and should therefore be routinely documented in clinical sleep study reports.

Respiratory failure

The development of hypercapnic respiratory failure in the setting of chronic obstructive pulmonary disease (COPD) is usually associated with SDB, such as OSAS or sleep-related hypoventilation. However, while OSAS is best treated with CPAP, sleep-related hypoventilation is probably best treated with non-invasive ventilatory support; long-term trials are under way to assess its effectiveness in this population. In the absence of primary pulmonary or cardiac disease, the development of hypercapnic respiratory failure may occur in extremely obese individuals (BMI > 40). In those with more modest obesity, OSAS is rarely a cause of hypercapnic respiratory failure.

Pulmonary hypertension

The relationship between OSAS and pulmonary artery hypertension remains tentative. Many studies investigating this issue have not controlled for underlying lung disease, such as COPD. However, in patients with OSAS in whom COPD is excluded, the prevalence of pulmonary arterial hypertension appears to be about 27%, and is more likely in heavier, more hypoxemic patients who have longer periods with oxygen saturations below 80%. Pulmonary artery pressures usually parallel hypercapnia and hypoventilation during sleep. During sleep, the mean pulmonary artery pressure can exceed 40 mmHg in patients with OSAS, but seldom reaches 25 mmHg when awake. In patients with OSAS and waking mean pulmonary artery pressures greater than 30 mmHg, additional causes of pulmonary hypertension should be sought (e.g. cardiac disease, thromboembolic disorders, vascular disease).

Gastroesophageal reflux

In normal individuals, silent reflux of gastric fluid is common during sleep. This fluid may be acidic or alkaline depending on acid release and medications (e.g. proton-pump inhibitors). When reflux becomes symptomatic, patients may awake with choking or laryngeal spasm; acid fluid in the esophagus is associated with vagal activity and bronchoconstriction.

The effects of gastroesophageal reflux are thought to be more pronounced in patients with OSAS. In one study, approximately two-thirds of OSAS patients complained of nocturnal reflux, and symptoms improved by about 50% when the apnea was treated with CPAP.

Mechanical factors induced by OSAS (negative intrathoracic and positive intra-abdominal pressures) may accentuate the movement of gastric fluid from the stomach to the esophagus. Patients with OSAS are commonly obese, and consume caffeine (to stay awake) and drink alcohol (to relax at night), all of which would further aggravate the reflux.

Preeclampsia

In recent years, snoring and OSAS have been recognized in pregnant women, particularly those with preeclampsia. Such mothers who snore and have apnea give birth to children of lower birth weight. In the mothers with hypertension, treatment of the apnea with CPAP may bring the systemic blood pressure down towards normal levels.

Glucose intolerance and other endocrine derangements

Although diabetes is not known to cause OSAS directly, it is recognized that conditions associated with neuropathy are likely to aggravate the disorder. Moreover, obesity is common feature of both diabetes mellitus and OSAS. In addition, OSAS is likely to aggravate diabetes mellitus, because elevated sympathetic nervous system activity related to untreated OSAS may contribute to a relative insulin resistance during sleep. Conversely, the work of breathing (and thus energy consumption) is greater in OSAS. When OSAS is treated, diabetic control may improve as a result of a reduction in circulating norepinephrine and improved insulin sensitivity.

An increased prevalence of OSAS has also been reported in patients with polycystic ovary syndrome, though the relationship is weakened when obesity is controlled for.

Difficult tracheal intubation

OSAS should be considered in any patient who is deemed difficult to intubate. Anesthesia care practitioners are in a prime position to observe the collapsibility of the upper airway, particularly immediately following extubation.

Observation of a crowded airway, which can be classified using the Mallampati score (Figure 3.3), predicts a difficult intubation.

Neurocognitive impairment

Neurocognitive impairment is one of the most important complications of OSAS and one of the most difficult to identify. Impairment can be divided into loss of higher mental function, reduced mood and excessive sleepiness.

Higher mental function. Detailed studies of brain function show that patients with OSAS have significant reductions in cerebral gray matter compared with those without apnea.

Patients with clinically diagnosed OSAS often have impaired cognitive function. Effective treatment has, however, been shown to improve some measures of cognitive function, even in those with

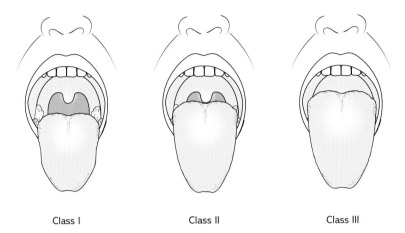

Class I   Class II   Class III

Figure 3.3 The Mallampati score is based on the appearance of the upper airway when the individual is awake, seated upright and saying 'Ahhh', without the use of a tongue depressor. In class I, the tip of the soft palate and the posterior pharyngeal wall can be easily visualized. In class II, the tip of the soft palate cannot be seen, though the posterior pharyngeal wall can still be visualized. In class III, none of the posterior pharyngeal wall can be seen. Adapted from Mallampati SR, Gatt SP, Gugino LD et al. A clinical sign to predict difficult tracheal intubation: a prospective study. *Can Anaesth Soc J* 1985;32(4):429–34.

mild OSAS, and is associated with improvements in attention, psychomotor speed, executive functioning and nonverbal delayed recall. There is some evidence that those patients with the greatest cognitive impairment, especially those with vigilance impairment, are more likely to comply with treatment for OSAS. Results from the SHHS showed no correlation between measures of OSAS and a small battery of cognitive function tests in a sample of about 1700 non-institutionalized individuals with mostly mild-to-moderate levels of OSAS. It is therefore likely that OSAS has an effect on cognition that is variable and interacts with other risk factors, such as age and socioeconomic status.

Mechanisms for cognitive impairment include:
• fragmented sleep
• loss of quality sleep (i.e. slow-wave and REM sleep)

- direct effects of hypoxemia and hypercapnia
- oscillations in blood pressure and cerebral flow.

The features of cognitive impairment can be quite subtle. Altered personality, inability to cope with stress, development of a 'short fuse' and reduced memory are common in OSAS.

Significant cognitive impairment has also been shown in children and medical students who snore compared with non-snoring control subjects. Children who snore perform worse at school and improve once snoring is treated (e.g. via tonsillectomy). OSAS has also been linked to attention deficit hyperactivity disorder in children, although work in this area is preliminary.

Mood disturbance. Whether mood disturbances (depression and anxiety) are related to OSAS remains to be confirmed, but they are indeed common in OSAS patients and can improve significantly with treatment for the disorder.

Excessive daytime sleepiness is the most important cognitive impairment and can be divided into sleepiness during passive (e.g. watching television, reading a book in bed, listening to music, sitting in front of a computer) and active situations (driving a car, operating heavy machinery, talking to someone). Excessive daytime sleepiness in active situations is clearly of great social importance given the potential for accidents. The ESS is a handy guide to measuring the degree of impairment (see page 17).

Accidents. A major concern relating to neurocognitive impairment is the predisposition of OSAS patients to accidents, including both driving mishaps and workplace accidents involving heavy equipment. A recent provocative article demonstrated that patients with OSAS have driving impairments of a similar magnitude to those who are intoxicated with alcohol. Patients with OSAS have an approximately threefold greater chance of having a motor vehicle accident (and up to twelvefold greater for single-vehicle accidents) compared with control subjects, but this increase in risk is obviated by treatment.

Accidents related to sleepiness occur in over one-third of rural accidents and in at least half of single-vehicle accidents. However, as other factors in addition to OSAS may contribute to sleepiness (commonly sleep deprivation and drug side effects), the terminology used to describe the cause of accidents is unclear.

Although OSAS appears to be a risk factor for automobile accidents, most drivers with OSAS do not have accidents. Trying to identify those at greatest risk is a current challenge. Not surprisingly, the risk of automobile accidents appears highest in those patients who report sleepiness while driving, and in those who have high ESS scores (> 11). Some recent evidence reveals that driving simulator technology may distinguish apneic drivers from other drivers, as well as those with apnea who are at less risk of automobile accidents. This same tool has demonstrated that driving capabilities improve to baseline levels when patients with OSAS are treated with nasal CPAP, and that this improvement may occur rapidly.

Quality of life and use of healthcare resources

Although it is difficult to control for comorbid medical conditions and obesity, OSAS is associated with reduced quality of life, which is improved by effective treatment with CPAP. Similarly, most studies have concluded that there is an association between OSAS and depressive symptoms, which improve when OSAS is treated. Furthermore, it is possible that untreated OSAS contributes to resistance to pharmacological treatment in some patients with mood disorders.

Data are now accumulating that patients with untreated OSAS make increased demands on healthcare resources, particularly for cardiovascular diseases and mood disorders. However, the use of healthcare resources is reduced in the year following diagnosis and initiation of treatment for OSAS compared with the year before diagnosis.

Finally, there is evidence that untreated OSAS results in shortened life expectancy. Several large studies controlling for obesity and other confounders have established that OSAS is a clear-cut risk factor for hypertension, car accidents, neurocognitive dysfunction and cardiovascular disease, including strokes. In addition, untreated OSAS is associated with reduced life expectancy, impaired quality of life, increased healthcare costs, glucose intolerance and even erectile dysfunction.

Physiological overview

Epidemiological and genetic studies indicate that the inheritance of OSAS is likely to be multigenic, and its development depends on environmental as well as genetic factors. A reduced airspace, usually (but not always) behind the uvula, leads to increased resistance to inspiratory airflow. Obesity further increases the work of breathing by causing abnormally high levels of negative pressure against the narrowed upper airway. This causes edema by suction, which is exacerbated by the trauma of snoring. If there is nasal obstruction (polyps, mucus, septal deviation), then increased *upstream* airway resistance increases the effects of the increased *downstream* negative pressure (intrathoracic vacuum). Hypertension and advancing age are additional common characteristics of patients with OSAS, and add to the morbidity of the condition.

Retrognathia, which results in posterior displacement of the tongue, also leads to posterior airway narrowing and may increase the risk of OSAS.

Cellular basis of cardiovascular disease. Individuals with OSAS have elevations in several biomarkers linked to cardiovascular risk, including C-reactive protein (CRP), leptin, homocysteine and insulin resistance.

CRP is an acute-phase reactant, which is increased in cell adhesion molecules. An elevated CRP level is associated with blunted endothelium-dependent vasodilation in resistance vessels and is correlated with an increased risk of developing cardiovascular disease. CRP is also correlated with the severity of OSAS, and this association of CRP and OSAS persists even when age, gender, BMI, smoking, alcohol consumption and cholesterol are controlled for.

Thus OSAS may cause endothelial dysfunction with CRP as one of the mediators.

Leptin is a protein secreted by fat cells, and is thought to be an appetite suppressant. Obese patients have high leptin levels and are believed to be resistant to appetite suppression mediated by leptin. However, both plasma leptin levels and historical weight gain are higher in OSAS patients than in weight-matched controls. Thus, OSAS may result in high leptin levels and enhanced leptin resistance, even beyond that which is 'normally' seen in obese individuals. Leptin has been identified as a promoter of platelet aggregation, and increased leptin levels are linked to hypertension, increased sympathetic activity and higher heart rate. In fact, leptin appears to be an independent and powerful predictor of cardiovascular events.

Homocysteine may cause endothelial dysfunction by promoting the progression of atherosclerosis. It increases oxidative stress and promotes vascular smooth muscle growth, and is emerging as an independent risk factor for cardiovascular disease. Patients with ischemic heart disease and OSAS have significantly higher homocysteine levels than patients who have only OSAS, patients who have OSAS and hypertension, and control subjects with neither OSAS nor heart disease. Hyperhomocysteinemia has been shown to be associated with hyperinsulinemia and may account, in part, for the increased risk of cardiovascular disease associated with hyperinsulinemia.

There are a variety of definitions of the metabolic syndrome, but all include some measure of obesity, hypertension, hyperlipidemia and insulin resistance. Although formal evidence of the prevalence of OSAS in patients with the metabolic syndrome is lacking, it is likely that there is a very high concordance and that OSAS is independently associated with insulin resistance. In fact, insulin resistance may be present in non-obese as well as obese individuals with OSAS. Insulin-resistance syndrome is an independent risk factor for cardiovascular disease.

Serum fibrinogen levels, tumor necrosis factor α, and interleukin-6 are also known to be risk factors for cardiovascular disease, and to be elevated in patients with OSAS. Circulating nitric oxide, which helps regulate vascular tone and may lower blood pressure, is reduced in patients with OSAS, but increased when these patients are treated effectively.

The findings of studies demonstrating that biomarkers of cardiovascular risk are increased in patients with OSAS are bolstered by burgeoning evidence demonstrating that OSAS is associated with hypertension, heart failure, cardiac ischemia and stroke.

Key points – medical complications of obstructive sleep apnea syndrome (OSAS)

- OSAS causes hypertension.
- OSAS is associated with congestive heart failure, cardiac arrhythmias and ischemic events.
- OSAS is associated with cognitive impairment and increased driving risk.
- OSAS is associated with mood disorders.
- OSAS is associated with increased use of healthcare resources.

Key references

Bassetti C, Aldrich MS. Sleep apnea in acute cerebrovascular diseases: final report on 128 patients. *Sleep* 1999;22:217–23.

Becker HF, Jerruntup A, Ploch T et al. Effect of nasal continuous positive airway pressure teatment on blood pressure in patients with obstructive sleep apnea. *Circulation* 2003;107:68–73.

Hack MA, Choi SJ, Vijayapalan P et al. Comparison of the effects of sleep deprivation, alcohol and obstructive sleep apnoea (OSA) on simulated steering performance. *Respir Med* 2001; 95:594–601.

He J, Kryger MH, Zorick FJ et al. Mortality and apnea index in obstructive sleep apnea; experience in 385 male patients. *Chest* 1988:94:9–14.

Ip MS, Lam B, Ng MM et al. Obstructive sleep apnea is independently associated with insulin resistance. *Am J Respir Crit Care Med* 2002;165:670–6.

Kaneko Y, Floras JS, Usui J et al. Cardiovascular effects of continuous positive airway pressure in patients with heart failure and obstructive sleep apnea. *N Engl J Med* 2003; 348:1233–41.

Nieto FJ, Young TB, Lind BK et al. Association of sleep-disordered breathing, sleep apnea, and hypertension in a large community-based study. *JAMA* 2000;283:1829–36.

Peker Y, Hedner J, Norum J et al. Increased incidence of cardiovascular disease in middle-aged men with obstructive sleep apnea. A 7-year follow-up. *Am J Respir Crit Care Med* 2002; 166:159–65.

Redline S, Strauss ME, Adams N et al. Neuropsychological function in mild sleep-disordered breathing. *Sleep* 1997;20:160–7.

Shahar E, Whitney CW, Redline S et al. Sleep-disordered breathing and cardiovascular disease. Cross-sectional results of the Sleep Heart Health Study. *Am J Respir Crit Care Med* 2001;163:19–25.

In-laboratory sleep testing, or polysomnography (PSG), is currently the standard diagnostic tool for OSAS. However, it is likely that the present emphasis on PSG alone, and particularly the AHI, will broaden in the future. Data are accumulating that the AHI is not an entirely sufficient measurement of OSAS, because it does not take into account how long the apneas or hypopneas last, the degree of sleep disturbance, the level of oxygen desaturation, or associated problems, such as cardiac arrhythmias. Furthermore, measures and definitions of SDB are not standardized; for example, some reports of SDB use definitions of hypopnea that require varying (or no) degrees of oxygen desaturation. There is also evidence that upper airway resistance syndrome (UARS) and even simple snoring can cause many of the sequelae of OSAS; PSG does not usually take this into account, and the sleep research community has been unable to convince most insurers to pay for treatment of these ill-defined forms of OSAS. Moreover, there remains an enormous debate about the cutoff between a 'normal' and an 'abnormal' AHI.

In addition to these problems, average waiting times for PSG in most countries are more than a month. With the increasing data to demonstrate that OSAS causes motor accidents, heart disease and death, physicians are becoming increasingly uncomfortable with letting patients wait weeks or months for testing, and then weeks or months before titration and definitive treatment. As a result, interest in and data on the usefulness of screening tools, clinical prediction formulas and portable or home monitoring are rapidly accumulating. It is therefore likely that these techniques will be increasingly used to triage those patients with obvious, severe OSAS to early treatment with autotitrating CPAP.

Definitions
The AHI is the criterion most commonly used to establish the diagnosis of OSAS and to quantify its severity (Table 4.1). Recently,

TABLE 4.1

Definitions

Apnea and hypopnea

Decrease in airflow or chest wall movement to an amplitude smaller than approximately 30% (apnea) or 70% (hypopnea) of baseline, lasting for at least 10 seconds. They are associated with oxyhemoglobin desaturation of $\geqslant$ 4% compared with baseline

Apnea–hypopnea index (AHI)

$$\frac{\text{Total number of episodes of apnea and hypopnea}}{\text{Total number of hours of sleep}}$$

Respiratory effort-related arousal (RERA)

A sequence of breaths characterized by increasing respiratory effort leading to an arousal from sleep which does not meet the criteria for an apnea or hypopnea. These events must fulfill both of the following criteria: a pattern of progressively more negative esophageal pressure, terminated by a sudden change in pressure to a less negative level; and an arousal. The event lasts 10 seconds or longer

Upper airways resistance syndrome (UARS)

A clinical syndrome of sleepiness resulting from respiratory effort-related arousals

Respiratory disturbance index (RDI)

Often used interchangeably with the apnea–hypopnea index, but may include respiratory effort-related arousals

Sleep-disordered breathing (SDB)

An ill-defined term used to encompass non-specific respiratory disturbances during sleep; may include snoring, asymptomatic apneas and full-blown obstructive sleep apnea syndrome

some unanimity in the criteria for defining apneas and hypopneas has been achieved, largely as a result of the SHHS. In adults, apneas and hypopneas require at least a 10-second reduction of airflow (to 30% of baseline for apneas and to 70% of baseline for hypopneas).

In the SHHS, the definitions of both apneas and hypopneas required an oxygen desaturation of 4% or more; notably, however, the definition of apnea promulgated by the American Academy of Sleep Medicine (AASM) and by the US Centers for Medicare and Medicaid Services (CMS, formerly the Health Care Financing Administration, HCFA) does not require oxygen desaturation (though the definition of hypopnea does). In obstructive apneas and hypopneas, reduction of airflow occurs despite continued ventilatory effort. In central apneas, respiratory effort is not detectable during the reduction in airflow.

According to the AASM, obstructive sleep apnea–hypopnea syndrome (OSAHS) exists when a patient has five or more obstructed breathing events per hour of sleep together with the appropriate clinical presentation.

In the USA, the CMS reimburse for CPAP treatment for patients with an AHI of more than 15, or an AHI of more than 5 in the presence of hypertension, stroke, sleepiness, ischemic heart disease or 'mood disorder'. Worldwide, however, there is extreme and evolving variability in the criteria used to initiate and pay for treatment. At the time of writing, in parts of Canada, CPAP will be covered based on the clinical judgment of a specialist without requirement for polysomnography. On the other hand, in Australia, extreme levels of SDB are required before treatment is publically funded.

Polysomnography

Overnight PSG remains the gold standard for the diagnosis of OSAS. A nocturnal PSG includes recordings of airflow, ventilatory effort, oxygen saturation, electrocardiogram, body position, electromyography (EMG) and electroencephalography (EEG). During a standard, laboratory-based PSG, a technician is present for the entire study to monitor the patient. A single overnight study is generally sufficient to diagnose OSAS; night-to-night variability in OSAS severity (as indicated by AHI) in the same person is approximately 10% and is thought to be due to changes in body position, alcohol consumption and other lifestyle factors.

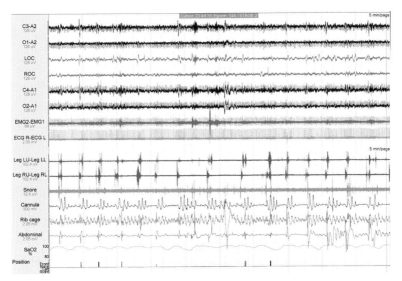

Figure 4.1 A 5-minute epoch from a polysomnogram showing salvos of obstructive events. C3-A2, O1-A2, C4-A1 and O2-A1, electroencephalogram leads; LOC and ROC, left and right oculogram; EMG, electromyogram; ECG, electrocardiogram; Leg LU and RU, left and right legs; Snore; Cannula, nasal pressure measurement; Rib cage and Abdominal, respective movement; SaO_2, oxygen saturation; Position, body position.

Often, SDB is sufficiently severe that the diagnosis of OSAS can be established early in the study (Figure 4.1). In this event, a 'split-night' study may be performed, where the second half of the study is used to titrate treatment (CPAP) for OSAS. In the USA, the CMS have recently endorsed split-night PSG, but have stipulated that the diagnostic portion of the test should last at least 2 hours to avoid artificially inflating the recorded severity of the SDB.

A normal overnight study makes significant OSAS very unlikely, but does not completely exclude it. Factors that may contribute to a false-negative sleep study include:

- poor-quality sleep during the study (particularly absence of REM sleep)
- sleeping in the lateral position instead of the usual supine sleeping position during the study (OSAS tends to be most severe in the supine position)

- omitting the usual alcohol or sedative agent on the night of the study
- insensitive (or, more accurately, overly sensitive) monitors of airflow and/or respiratory effort, which allow subtle decrements in airflow and/or marked increases in respiratory effort to go undetected.

Recording techniques. Although there is now some consistency in the definitions used for OSAS, considerable variations remain in recording techniques for measures of airflow and respiratory effort. Pneumotachography and esophageal manometry are the most accurate measures of airflow and respiratory effort, respectively, but are rarely used clinically because they are cumbersome. Thermistry, which relies on a qualitative signal to make quantitative inferences about airflow, is probably the most commonly used technique to assess breathing in clinical sleep laboratories. The use of a pressure transducer as a means of assessing nasal airflow is more accurate than thermistry, and will probably supplant it. In the meantime, the innate inaccuracy and variability of current measurement techniques have almost certainly resulted in varying sensitivity for detection of OSAS.

Upper airways resistance syndrome

One probable consequence of lack of standardized definitions and measurement techniques for OSAS is the confusion and controversy surrounding UARS. UARS is characterized by increased respiratory efforts with frequent arousals, but without overt apneas or reductions in airflow. This fragmented sleep pattern results in increased daytime sleepiness and an abnormally short latency on the Multiple Sleep Latency Test. In the original description of UARS, increased respiratory effort was detected by esophageal pressure nadirs that were more negative than one standard deviation below the mean, followed by transient EEG arousals. These arousals were termed respiratory effort-related arousals (RERA). A recent AASM panel defined a RERA event as 'A sequence of breaths characterized by increasing respiratory effort leading to an arousal from sleep, but which does not meet criteria for an apnea or hypopnea'.

Techniques currently used to detect UARS in sleep laboratories vary greatly, but few clinical centers actually measure UARS in accordance with its original definition. Since there is no clear standard for diagnosing for this condition, it is probably both under- and overdiagnosed. Although there is clearly some variability in the measurement and consequences of UARS, some individuals who do not meet the classic criteria for OSAS work so hard to breathe at night that their sleep is nonrefreshing.

Prediction formulas

Several investigators have developed formulas for predicting OSAS based on the history or physical examination. Among the most useful findings are a history of witnessed apneas, male gender, BMI and neck circumference. In general, these formulas are sensitive but non-specific compared with PSG. While there is growing evidence that 'classic' sleep apneics (i.e. sicker, heavier, male) can be diagnosed clinically without formal laboratory PSG, there are many patients who do not fit the stereotypical prototype of the obstructive sleep apneic. These include Asians, women and older individuals. Nevertheless, prediction formulas probably do have a place in the expedited diagnosis and/or triage of patients with suspected OSAS, despite the fact that they are not currently recognized by most third-party payers in the USA.

A novel prediction formula to identify OSAS is based on neck circumference and the presence or absence of snoring, systemic hypertension and nocturnal choking. The formula can be used for patients with neck circumferences of more than 40 cm in women and 43 cm in men. A point score is added to the neck circumference measured in centimeters for snoring (+3), hypertension (+4) and nocturnal choking (+3). Thus a male with a neck circumference of 45 cm who snores would have a score of 48 (45 + 3) and, if he was also hypertensive, he would have a score of 52 (45 + 3 + 4). A clinical probability of OSAS can then be assigned based on the total score: below 43 represents a low probability; 43–48 a moderate probability; and over 48 a high probability. In such a model, a simplified diagnostic tool (limited channel or split-night study) can then be used to assess patients with a low or high probability, whereas those with a moderate probability would undergo full PSG.

Ambulatory monitoring

Controversy exists as to the best place to perform sleep studies and about the role of screening. Proponents of home testing suggest that it has the benefits of enhanced patient convenience, reduced cost and increased accessibility. Opponents point out that, with home studies, split-night studies cannot be done, equipment problems cannot be corrected, 'live' assessments cannot be made and non-OSAS disorders cannot be detected. However, the best data about the consequences and definitions of OSAS actually come from portable monitoring. Ambulatory monitoring, which can measure as many channels as laboratory PSG, was used in the SHHS. The SHHS, using rigid protocols and a central reading system, demonstrated that home monitoring can produce reliable data with acceptable rates of data loss.

In clinical situations, however, home monitoring may not be so advantageous. It has not yet been shown to reduce the cost of diagnosis of OSAS, and is not uniformly reimbursed in the USA. Furthermore, possibly because of the resources already invested in 'full-service' sleep laboratories, those working in sleep medicine have been slow to utilize the new data on home monitoring that has emerged from the SHHS and other research.

Oximetry

Oximetry is obviously the basis for the current definitions of OSAS. In general, patients with significant OSAS have greater fluctuations in oxygen saturation (and heart rate) than those without apnea (Figure 4.2). However, thinner, younger patients without lung disease can have significant breathing and sleep disturbance without remarkable oxygen desaturation. Furthermore, patients with underlying lung disease may have oxygen desaturation without OSAS. Thus, oximetry is neither sensitive nor specific for OSAS.

(a)

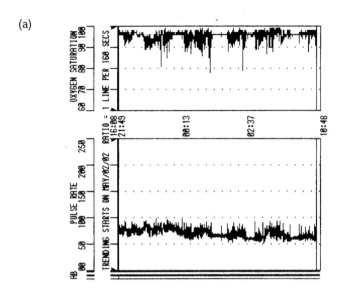

(b)

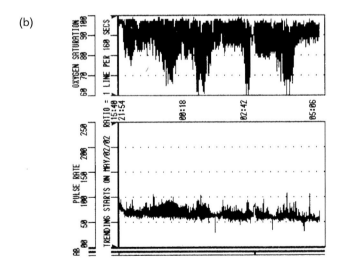

Figure 4.2 Continuous oximetry and heart rate measurements in two patients.

(a) A patient with moderately severe obstructive sleep apnea syndrome.

(b) A patient with severe obstructive sleep apnea syndrome. Both patients had a high pretest probability of having obstructive sleep apnea syndrome (they were both obese, snorers, and had witnessed apneas and systemic hypertension).

47

Studies that have investigated oximetry as a screening or diagnostic tool for OSAS have drawn conflicting conclusions. Although oximetry has been reported to be a valid diagnostic tool in the UK, it has generally not been endorsed in the USA.

Oximeter sampling times are critical to diagnostic accuracy for OSAS, but are often overlooked. Ideally, the sampling (averaging) rate should be about 2 seconds; if the sampling interval is too long (e.g. > 5 seconds), sensitivity for OSA events is reduced. Clearly, this is not just an issue for oximetry as a screening tool, but also for in-laboratory PSG, since measures of OSAS are highly dependent on changes in oxygen saturation. Thus, with improved sampling times and sensitivity, the technique may prove acceptable for large population screening studies once further studies are completed.

Other tools

Several other tools have been developed to aid in the diagnosis or screening of OSAS. Although currently not accepted by mainstream sleep specialists, these techniques do have a physiological basis and some diagnostic utility. They include measures of movement, such as actigraphy and static beds assessment. Also being developed, particularly by cardiologists, are measures of heart rate variability and pulse pressure, including holter monitoring.

Key points – diagnosis

- Polysomnography is the current gold standard for the diagnosis of obstructive sleep apnea syndrome, but it does have several pitfalls.
- Clinical prediction formulas can exclude obstructive sleep apnea syndrome with a fair degree of accuracy.
- Oximetry is a useful screening and diagnostic tool.

Key references

American Academy of Sleep Medicine Task Force. Sleep-related breathing disorders in adults: Recommendations for syndrome definition and measurement techniques in clinical research. *Sleep* 1999; 22: 667–89.

Davila DG, Richards KC, Marshall BL et al. Oximeter's acquisition parameter influences the profile of respiratory disturbances. *Sleep* 2003;26:91–5.

Flemons WW, Whitelaw WA, Brant R, Remmers JE. Likelihood ratios for a sleep apnea prediction rule. *Am J Respir Crit Care Med* 1994;150: 1279–85.

Golpe R, Jimenez A, Carpizo R. Home sleep studies in the assessment of sleep apnea/hypopnea syndrome. *Chest* 2002;122:1156–61.

Guilleminault C, Stoohs R, Clerk A et al. A cause of excessive daytime sleepiness. The upper airway resistance syndrome. *Chest* 1993;104: 781–7.

Kushida CA, Efron B, Guilleminault C. A predictive morphometric model for the obstructive sleep apnea syndrome. *Ann Intern Med* 1997;127:581–7.

Maislin G, Pack AI, Kribbs NB et al. A survey screen for prediction of apnea. *Sleep* 1995;18:158–66.

Meoli AL, Casey KR, Clark RW, and the Clinical Practice Review Committee of the American Academy of Sleep Medicine. Hypopnea in sleep-disordered breathing in adults. *Sleep* 2001;24:469–70.

Netzer NC, Stoohs RA, Netzer CM et al. Using the Berlin Questionnaire to identify patients at risk for the sleep apnea syndrome. *Ann Intern Med* 1999;131:485–91.

Quan SF, Griswold ME, Iber C et al. for the Sleep Heart Health Study (SHHS) Research Group. Short-term variability of respiration and sleep during unattended nonlaboratory polysomnography – the Sleep Heart Health Study. *Sleep* 2002;25:843–9.

Rowley JA, Aboussouan LS, Badr S. The use of clinical prediction formulae in the evaluation of obstructive sleep apnea. *Sleep* 2000;23:929–38.

The most successful medical management of OSAS relies on the use of positive airway pressure and of oral appliances. Other strategies to reduce the severity of OSAS are also covered in this chapter and include a review of medication and social drug use, weight loss and changes in sleep habits.

Positive airway pressure

Positive airway pressure maintains upper airway patency during sleep simply by providing a pneumatic splint. It leads to improvements in quality of life, mood and alertness in patients with OSAS. Recent advances in masks, humidification, pressure delivery systems and patient education have improved adherence to treatment.

Masks have developed from simple molded pieces of silicone into a variety of cushions, some with flexible foam and others with single- or double-layered silicone (Figure 5.1). Masks can be nasal, nasal prong (or 'pillows'), oral or oronasal ('full-face'). Although clinicians and patients have definite preferences, only the nasal pillow type has been shown to increase compliance. The exhalation ports are an important part of the mask system and enable a continuous bias flow of exhaled air to prevent rebreathing. Generally, nasal masks are most popular and best tolerated.

Oral masks are useful in patients who have intractable nasal obstruction and in those in whom nasal positive airway pressure should be avoided (e.g. immediately after nasal surgery, or following trans-sphenoidal pituitary surgery, associated with a fractured base of skull). Orally delivered positive airway pressure requires humidification (see below) as the normal humidification process provided by the nose is bypassed.

Oronasal or full-face masks are best used by patients with intractable leakage (usually a nasal mask with oral leakage). Such

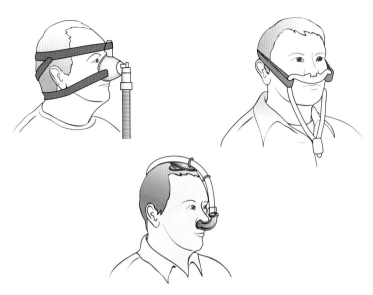

Figure 5.1 A variety of continuous positive airway pressure (CPAP) masks are available. Although CPAP masks typically fit over the nose, they can also fit over the nose and the mouth (full-face masks). Nasal pillow interfaces are for tight-fitting prongs that insert directly into the nostrils. Masks can be made from a variety of substances, including soft acrylic or acrylic-covered foam or gel.

masks are commonly used in patients with acute respiratory failure (e.g. congestive heart failure or chronic obstructive lung disease), many of whom may require long-term positive airway pressure.

Masks should be cleaned with warm soapy water daily to reduce the amount of facial oil adhering to the mask, and thus reduce the chance of air leakage.

Pressure. Positive airway pressure can be delivered by an electric flow generator in a number of ways.

Continuous positive airway pressure (CPAP) is a constant pressure, usually 5–20 cmH$_2$O, throughout the respiratory cycle. Treatment is usually started during PSG in a sleep laboratory. It is the type of therapy that is most commonly used and reported in clinical intervention trials. The great majority of patients do well with 8–10 cmH$_2$O pressure.

Bilevel positive airway pressure provides a greater inspiratory pressure and lower expiratory pressure. It was initially developed to assist ventilation in patients with hypercapnic respiratory failure, but trials have been carried out in patients with OSAS. However, in the small studies in OSAS patients reported so far, there is no convincing improvement in well-being or compliance with treatment with bilevel positive airway pressure compared with CPAP.

Cflex. Recently, a modification of bilevel positive airway pressure called Cflex has been developed in which the expiratory pressure is 1–4 cmH$_2$O lower than the inspiratory pressure. Clinical trials to determine whether Cflex offers any advantage over CPAP are pending.

Autotitrating (or 'smart') CPAP is a system in which a variable pressure is delivered at a level determined by computerized algorithms within the flow generator, based on the pump sensing flow limitation and snoring. Such devices may improve patient comfort and tolerability. Patients who require a large difference in pressure to prevent snoring (e.g. because of the effects of posture or sleep stage), those on high levels of standard CPAP (i.e. > 10 cmH$_2$O) and those with adverse effects from excessive pressure (dry throat or rhinitis) are the groups most likely to benefit from autotitrating positive airway pressure. These devices achieve a reduction of about 2 cmH$_2$O in the delivered mean positive airway pressure compared with standard CPAP devices. The computer technology included in the system can also store details of ventilation over days to weeks, and can thus provide detailed adherence data (such as leak). Compliance with autotitrating CPAP may be better than that with standard CPAP; however, early evidence also suggests that not all autotitrating CPAP machines are equally effective.

Compliance. Most devices now come with an hour meter (also known as a compliance meter) that monitors 'machine on' or 'mask on' time, allowing the clinician to assess the patient's compliance with treatment. It is now generally accepted that the aim should be treatment for more than 7 hours/night to ensure maximal resolution of OSAS signs and symptoms; however, one arbitrary definition of adequate compliance is the use of CPAP for 4 or more hours on 5 or more nights/week.

Motivated patients will go to great lengths to avoid discomfort and ensure that CPAP works (Figure 5.2).

Humidification. Most people using nasal CPAP occasionally leak air through their mouths when asleep. This can lead to symptoms of dry mouth and nose, and troublesome rhinitis may ensue, making patients reluctant to use positive airway pressure. The addition of a humidifier may, however, augment comfort levels and thus adherence to treatment.

Humidification is usually delivered using a heated pass-over device sufficient to increase the relative humidity from 60% to 81% with the mouth closed, and from 43% to 64% with mouth leak. Heated humidification with a full-face mask maintains relative

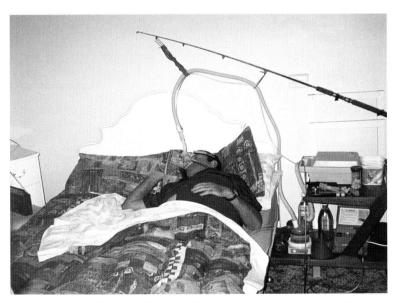

Figure 5.2 Discomfort may affect compliance, but can be overcome: in this case, a patient with severe hypercapnic emphysema devised a support for the tubing of his nasally delivered bilevel positive airway pressure treatment mask.

humidity at about 80% with or without mouth leak, and is often used for patients with intractable rhinitis. Cold-water pass-over humidifiers are also available, but do little to increase humidity unless the environmental air is extremely dry (e.g. in aircraft).

Humidifiers usually require cold boiled or distilled water. Nevertheless, daily emptying and cleaning of the humidifier device is recommended to prevent secondary microbial infection.

Complications and side effects of positive airway pressure.
Significant or life-threatening complications of positive airway pressure are extremely rare. Barotrauma is extremely improbable as, at high pressures, the mask system is likely to become dislodged or mouth leak will occur (with nasal masks); there are no convincing reports in the literature.

Rhinitis commonly occurs and can be dealt with by reducing the pressure, adding humidification, using an oronasal mask, a trial of autotitrating CPAP or nasal steroids. Nasal hemorrhage, though uncommon, does occur and should be treated according to the nasal pathology; humidification should be considered.

Pneumoencephalus is an unusual, but important, complication to recognize. It usually occurs in a patient who has previously suffered a fracture at the base of skull with a persistent connection between the nasal and cranial vaults that allows pressurized air to enter the skull. Such patients should cease treatment via the nasal route immediately. Oral positive airway pressure or tracheostomy should be considered as alternatives.

Conjunctivitis can occur if there is leak around the bridge of the nose. If the leak occurs during sleep and the patient is unaware of it until the morning, it can cause corneal damage. Fortunately, this is rare, as most people find conjunctival irritation so annoying that it wakes them up.

A poorly fitting mask can cause skin abrasions. The most important problem is damage to the skin across the bridge of the nose, which can become ulcerated and lead to cellulitis if not cared for adequately (Figure 5.3). Some patients keep two or more masks to alter the pressure placed on the facial skin. Allergy to the masks

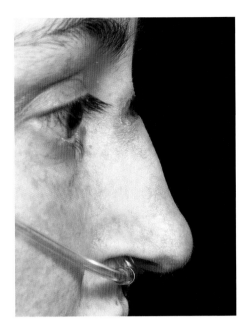

Figure 5.3 A young woman developed an ulcer over the bridge of her nose as a result of a poorly fitting mask, pulled too tight and left in place for > 48 hours over a weekend following an admission for acute respiratory failure.

is extremely uncommon; latex (a common skin allergen for healthcare workers) is not used in the preparation of most masks.

Oral appliances

Tongue protrusion devices work by pulling the tongue forward using a variety of methods, including simple suction with a bulb suction device. These devices are not, however, particularly successful.

Mandibular advancement splints have been the most successful oral devices used (Figure 5.4). Splints are available as single-piece, two-piece or adjustable devices; over 80 varieties of antisnoring oral splints exist! Although the improvement achieved with these splints is less than that seen with positive airway pressure, with careful patient selection about 50% of patients achieve a 50% reduction in AHI. It is, however, important that the splint maintains the mouth in a closed position during sleep.

Before fitting a splint, a lateral cephalogram and orthopantomography (OPG) may assist in determining mechanical

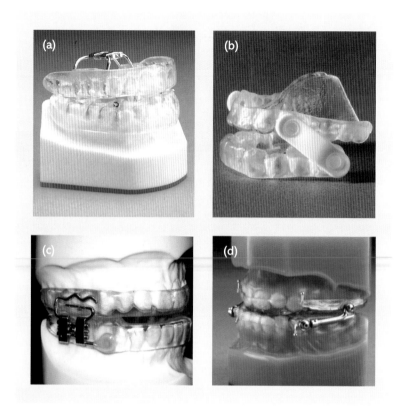

Figure 5.4 Examples of mandibular advancement splints. (a) Klearway; (b) EMA; (c) PM2; (d) Herbst. Images courtesy of (a) Professor Alan A Lowe DMD, University of British Columbia; (b) Frantz Design Inc.; (c, d) Professor Donald Falace DMD, University of Kentucky College of Dentistry.

or dental contraindications. These include temporomandibular joint pain, poor/missing dentition, gum disease and nasal obstruction. In addition, patients with chronic pain or myalgia and anxiety generally do not tolerate mandibular splints well.

Side effects of wearing a splint include gum or tooth pain and excessive salivation. Long-term adherence to a dental splint is about 50% at 6 months. This form of treatment is most suited to patients with mild-to-moderate OSAS and to snorers. In a recent trial, oral appliances were shown to be more effective in the treatment of OSAS than uvulopalatopharyngoplasty.

Maxillary expansion. The novel observation of OSAS in patients with Marfan's syndrome led a group of researchers to assess the effects of a high arched palate on the condition. A narrow and high arched palate was thought to contribute to OSAS by creating a small nasal space, and thus elevated nasal resistance, and causing the tongue to be positioned both inferiorly and posteriorly. Patients with Marfan's syndrome also have reduced compliance of collagen tissue in and around the oropharynx.

Even in the absence of Marfan's syndrome, many patients with OSAS will be found to have a narrow maxillary width and may benefit from maxillary expansion. In children, this may be achieved simply by wearing a mouth splint and gradually expanding the maxillae. In adults, it may be necessary to split the hard palate surgically and then use a splint to maintain the separation until new bone forms. Occasionally, repositioning of the front teeth is required after maxillary expansion.

Medications to avoid

It is important to avoid some medications that might exacerbate OSAS, such as glucocorticoids, narcotics, codeine, sedatives, muscle relaxants and antiepileptics. In addition, muscle relaxants, including alcohol and sleeping pills, can make apneas longer by reducing airway tone and by increasing the arousal threshold.

Potentially useful medications

The role of tricyclic antidepressants and serotonin reuptake inhibitors in controlling OSAS has been investigated. However, initial partial success in uncontrolled trials could not be confirmed in controlled trials.

In men, progesterone may reduce AHI and improve daytime oxygen saturation, but the side effects (thromboembolic risk and reduced libido) are generally unacceptable. However, a large cross-sectional study of postmenopausal women showed that OSAS was less common in those who took hormone replacement therapy (HRT) than in those who did not, and one very small interventional study suggested that HRT may improve OSAS in postmenopausal women.

Nasal steroids can reduce snoring. They have also been shown to reduce the AHI in both children and adults. In addition, they are useful in the treatment of vasomotor rhinitis associated with CPAP.

Inhaled surfactant may alter the surface tension of the upper airway, and thus make it less likely to collapse. Unfortunately, high cost and short half-life limit the usefulness of this unique potential treatment.

One small study of the use of proton-pump inhibitors in patients with fairly severe OSAS showed improvement (but not normalization) of the respiratory disturbance index.

Social drugs

Cigarette smoking increases the severity of OSAS, probably by increasing nasal resistance. In addition, nicotine disrupts sleep. In general, smokers have more sleep disturbances than non-smokers. Smoking cessation advice and support should be part of the routine management of all patients who smoke.

Alcohol consumption should also be minimized or avoided as alcohol relaxes the muscles of the upper airway (it loosens the tongue while awake and asleep!), increases nasal resistance (via vasodilatation) and delays brainstem recognition of disturbed ventilation.

Sleep quantity

Loss of sleep (i.e. sleep deprivation) is associated with impaired upper airway muscle activity in response to rising levels of carbon dioxide; thus, protective factors, such as upper airway dilating muscle strength, may be lost with sleep deprivation. Good sleep hygiene or habits should be discussed and promoted among patients with OSAS (Table 6.1).

Sleep position

A subset of patients (usually those who are thinner, older and with milder disease) may have position-dependent apnea. In these individuals, sleeping on the side may totally eliminate OSAS.

TABLE 5.1

Sleep hygiene

- Sleep only when sleepy
- If you cannot fall asleep within 20 minutes, get up and do something boring until you feel sleepy
- Do not take naps
- Get up and go to bed at the same time every day
- Refrain from exercise at least 4 hours before bedtime
- Develop sleep rituals
- Use your bed for sleeping and sex only
- Stay away from caffeine, nicotine and alcohol for at least 4–6 hours before you go to bed
- Make sure your bed and bedroom are quiet, cool and comfortable
- Use sunlight and physical activity to set your biological clock

Generally, avoiding sleeping in the supine position will reduce apnea. The difficulty is in keeping the body in a non-supine position; options include sewing a small object or even a tennis ball inside the pajama coat or placing a pillow under the middle of the mattress. However, most clinicians are uncomfortable treating a condition known to have serious cardiovascular and public health consequences using this technique.

Patients occasionally find that sleeping on two or three pillows also helps attenuate the sound of snoring. Some patients with severe OSAS sleep upright in a recliner; this approach helps to keep the tongue and jaw from falling back and occluding the airway, but should be considered 'first aid' at best.

Weight loss

Weight gain and the development of obesity is associated with increased neck circumference and fat deposited in the lateral walls of the upper airway. The shape of the upper airway and the composition of the walls changes in obesity. The relationship between weight, sleep and appetite is complex, and probably mediated in part by leptin, cortisol, insulin and metabolic rate. Patients with newly diagnosed OSAS have a greater increase in weight in the year before diagnosis than their weight-matched controls, and patients who comply with CPAP tend to gain weight though it is not known why. Leptin, a hormone released in response to obesity, may reduce the ventilatory response and thus prolong episodes of apnea and hypopnea. The development of OSAS further aggravates other cardiovascular-related illnesses (e.g. diabetes, hypertension). In one study, a 10% reduction in body weight was associated with a 26% reduction in the AHI.

All obese patients with OSAS should be counseled about weight loss. Unfortunately, weight loss takes time and is maintained in only a minority of patients. Patients are confused about fat grams, 'sugar busters', exercise expenditure, liquid diets and bariatric surgery. In the long run, simple advice about calorie intake and output may be most effective. The two pharmacological approaches to weight loss that are still available in the USA have respectable long-term (2 year) results of 8–10%. A commercially available program, Weight Watchers, has now been shown to promote and maintain weight loss more effectively than a 'self-help' approach. A recent review advises clinicians to assume that patients who are obese know that they are, establish a specific plan, identify any barriers, ensure follow-up and avoid criticism.

Relieving nasal obstruction

Nasal resistance can be reduced by removing allergens, including cigarette smoke and common allergens such as house dust mite and animal dander, and avoiding alcohol. Nasal steroid sprays and decongestants may help in the short term. Nasal dilator strips can also be helpful. Occasionally, surgical clearance of the nasal passages (e.g. inferior turbinectomy, submucosal resection, polypectomy) may reduce snoring.

Breastfeeding

Prevention is likely to be the most cost-effective way to control the incidence of OSAS. Breast-feeding an infant for a period of more

---

Key points – medical management

- Continuous positive airway pressure (CPAP) is the safest, cheapest, most effective and best-studied treatment for OSAS.
- CPAP compliance remains a clinical challenge, but attention to mask fit and comfort, humidity and keeping the nose unobstructed can help.
- Oral appliances, which are usually made by dentists, are useful for mild obstructive sleep apnea syndrome and for snoring.
- Weight loss can be curative in mild obstructive sleep apnea syndrome, and can reduce severity of more severe obstructive sleep apnea syndrome. It is rarely accomplished.
- Alcohol, cigarettes and sleep deprivation worsen sleep-disordered breathing, and should be discouraged.
- Nasal corticosteroids can reduce the apnea–hypopnea index, and can help with allergic nasal congestion and with vasomotor rhinitis associated with continuous positive airway pressure.
- Some patients have obstructive sleep apnea syndrome that is worsened or occurs exclusively when they are supine. Methods to achieve the lateral sleeping position are, however, fairly unsophisticated.
- Oxygen administration may normalize hypoxemia, but does not prevent sleep disruption and does not reverse daytime sleepiness, so it is only partially effective.

---

than 3 months, and up to 12 months if possible, is likely to improve the placement of the facial bones. The muscles required to breastfeed may place beneficial strains on the bony structure of the face and allow a more normal bony upper airway to develop. (Bottle-fed babies use different muscles, which produce different strains on the bony structure, and develop a narrower and more bony upper airway.) Breastfeeding also prevents the development of obesity and diabetes, which are known to exacerbate OSAS.

Supplemental oxygen

OSAS is a disorder of mechanical obstruction to the upper airway, and no increase in the concentration of inspired oxygen will maintain the airway. Oxygen is, therefore, reserved for patients with intrinsic lung disease, such as COPD. Studies comparing oxygen with CPAP in patients with OSAS have that both approaches improve sleep, cognition and some cardiovascular measures, but only CPAP improves daytime sleepiness.

An additional group that might benefit from oxygen are those with CSA (Cheyne–Stokes respiration). In these patients, supplemental oxygen may stabilize ventilation, probably through the mechanism of hypercapnia.

Key references

Foster GD. Principles and practices in the management of obesity. *Am J Respir Crit Care Med* 2003;168:274–80.

Farre R, Montserrat JM, Rigau J et al. Response of automatic continuous positive airway pressure devices to different sleep breathing patterns: a bench study. *Am J Respir Crit Care Med* 2002;166:469.

Flemons WW. Obstructive sleep apnea. *N Engl J Med* 2002;347: 498–504.

Fritsch KM, Iseli A, Russi EW, Bloch KE. Side effects of mandibular advancement devices for sleep apnea treatment. *Am J Respir Crit Care Med* 2001; 164:813–8.

Gotsopoulos H, Chen C, Qian J, Cistulli PA. Oral appliance therapy improves symptoms in obstructive sleep apnea: a randomized controlled trial. *Am J Respir Crit Care Med* 2002;177:743–8.

Hudgel DW, Thanakitcharu S. Pharmacologic treatment of sleep-disordered breathing. *Am J Respir Crit Care Med* 1999;158:691–9.

Kiely JL, Nolan P, McNicholas WT. Intranasal corticosteroid therapy for sleep apnoea in patients with co-existing rhinitis. *Thorax* 2004;59:50–5.

Martins de Araujo MT, Viera SB, Vasquez EC, Fleury B. Heated humidification or face mask to prevent upper airway dryness during continuous positive airway pressure therapy. *Chest* 2000;117:142–7.

Massie CA, Hart RW, Peralez K, Richards GN. Effects of humidification on nasal symptoms and compliance in sleep apnea patients using continuous positive airway pressure. *Chest* 1999;116: 403–8.

McArdle N, Devereux G, Heidarnejad H et al. Long-term use of CPAP therapy for sleep apnea/hypopnea syndrome. *Am J Respir Crit Care Med* 1999; 159:1108.

McEvoy RD, Sharp DJ, Thornton AT. The effects of posture on obstructive sleep apnea. *Am Rev Resp Dis* 1986;133:662–6.

Peppard PE, Young T, Palta M et al. Longitudinal study of moderate weight change and sleep disordered breathing. *JAMA* 2000;284:3015–21.

Teschler H, Wessendorf TE, Farhat AA et al. Two months auto-adjusting versus conventional nCPAP for obstructive sleep apnea syndrome. *Eur Resp J* 2000; 15:990.

A variety of surgical approaches have been used for OSAS, including tracheostomy, uvulopalatopharyngoplasty (UPPP), septoplasty, oromaxillofacial surgery and radiofrequency volumetric tissue reduction (RFVTR). In general, however, these approaches have been poorly evaluated, and data on long-term follow-up and the effects on automobile accidents, quality of life, blood pressure, cognitive performance and health care costs are lacking.

Uvulopalatopharyngoplasty

UPPP is the most commonly performed and best studied of the surgical procedures used for OSAS (Figure 7.1). It has a success rate of approximately 50% and appears to be even less effective in sicker, heavier patients. In particular, outcomes are poorer for those with a BMI over 30 or an oxygen saturation below 88%. Relapse

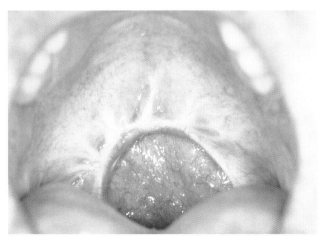

Figure 7.1 The appearance of the palate in a patient who had undergone uvulopalatopharyngoplasty (UPPP), but developed an infection and hemorrhage postoperatively. He recovered, but was left with severe fibrosis and loss of tissue compliance around the site of the UPPP. He also developed severe nasopharyngeal escape of food and liquids.

also occurs in those who respond and is usually related to weight gain. A recent comparison between UPPP and oral appliances for the treatment of OSAS found that oral appliances had better long-term and short-term outcomes.

Non-invasive techniques (e.g. laser-assisted UPPP) have not been well-evaluated, but appear to be less successful than invasive UPPP.

Radiofrequency volumetric tissue reduction

RFVTR of the palate (somnoplasty) has recently been described as a treatment for OSAS. The technique appears to be safe and less painful than laser-assisted UPPP, but has been used primarily for snoring, rather than for significant OSAS.

Oromaxillofacial surgery

Oromaxillofacial surgery is performed in very few centers, and the outcome in the long term has not been well-evaluated. A recent meta-analysis by Prinsell concludes that maxillomandibular advancement surgery for OSAS 'is a highly successful and potentially definitive primary single-staged surgery that may result in a significant reduction in OSAS-related health risks, as well as financial savings for the health care system'. However, 'successful' surgery was defined variously, but typically included patients with AHIs in the range of 10–20, which would still be considered pathological OSAS by most clinicians. Furthermore, the criteria for AHI were not cited anywhere in the article. Data on important outcomes, such as car accidents, cardiac function, cognitive function, quality of life and operative complications, are scarce. Long-term outcome data are nonexistent. Maxillomandibular advancement may be of benefit to carefully selected (thin) patients, who cannot or will not accept CPAP and who are willing to accept the risk of a procedure for which the short-term efficacy appears modest and the long-term efficacy and consequences are unknown.

Tracheostomy

Tracheostomy remains the gold-standard approach to severe OSAS in those who are intolerant of CPAP and are at immediate risk.

There are, however, problems associated with tracheostomy: loss of humidification, inability to cough and difficulty preventing water entering the trachea when bathing.

Gastric bariatric surgery

Gastric bariatric surgery has a place in the surgical management of OSAS, given the strong relationship between OSAS and obesity. Laparoscopic gastric-banding surgery is a relatively safe procedure that enables significant weight loss to be achieved. Overall, the BMI falls from about 40 to 30. Complications of gastroesophageal reflux disease and nutritional deficiency can be minimized by careful preoperative selection and close postoperative monitoring.

Key points – surgery

- Uvulopalatopharyngoplasty, the best-studied of all surgical approaches to treat obstructive sleep apnea syndrome, has a success rate of about 50% and a high relapse rate.
- Oromaxillofacial surgery may benefit carefully selected patients, but is not well-studied at present.
- Tracheostomy is the 'gold standard' surgical treatment for obstructive sleep apnea syndrome.
- Bariatric surgery shows promise as a treatment for obstructive sleep apnea syndrome.

Key references

Larsson LH, Carlsson-Norlander B, Svanbord E. Four-year follow-up after uvulopalatopharyngo-plasty in 50 unselected patients with obstructive sleep apnea syndrome. *Laryngoscope* 1994;104:1362–8.

Li KK, Powell NB, Riley RW, Guilleminault C. Temperature-controlled radiofrequency tongue base reduction for sleep-disordered breathing: long-term outcomes. *Otolaryngol Head Neck Surg* 2002;127:230–4

Prinsell JR. Maxillomandibular advancement surgery for obstructive sleep apnea syndrome. *J Am Dent Assoc* 2002;133:1489–97.

Sher AE. Upper airway surgery for obstructive sleep apnea. *Sleep Med Rev* 2002;6:195–212.

Thatcher GW, Maisel RH. The long-term evaluation of tracheostomy in the management of severe obstructive sleep apnea. *Laryngoscope* 2003;113:201–4.

Walker-Engstrom ML, Tegelberg A, Wilhelmsson B, Ringqvist I. 4-year follow up of treatment with dental appliance or uvulopalatopharyngoplasty in patients with obstructive sleep apnea: a randomized study. *Chest* 2002;121:739–46.

Epidemiology

Both the true prevalence and the recognition of OSAS will increase as the population becomes older and more obese. It is likely that attention will focus on OSAS at each end of the age spectrum, especially since it is associated with learning deficits and cognitive dysfunction, which are important in the young and old, respectively.

The genetic basis of OSAS is likely to become more firmly established, particularly in populations that are not typically obese, such as Asians.

Strong associations between OSAS and cardiovascular disease will continue to emerge, as will further evidence that OSAS is a public health problem, both because of its prevalence as well as the fact that it endangers others. Attention will be drawn to other disorders in which OSAS is very likely, but usually not considered, such as disorders of intellectual capacity (e.g. Down's syndrome), and endocrine (hypothyroidism, diabetes mellitus, acromegaly), cardiac and neurological disorders. It will, however, be necessary to overcome the desire of clinicians to treat conditions pharmacologically rather than physically with devices, such as CPAP.

Diagnosis

Approximately 10% of suspected OSAS patients have been diagnosed; thus more work is required to diagnose and treat the prevalence before new cases (incidence) are dealt with.

The current standard method of diagnosis, PSG, is expensive, cumbersome and time-consuming, while the indications for its use are widening (e.g. hypertension, preeclampsia, nocturia, sleepiness) and the therapeutic implications are staggering (e.g. the role of CPAP in heart failure). A simplified, more streamlined approach to diagnosis is therefore required. This may come in the form of risk stratification based on the history and physical examination followed by a simplified, combined, highly sensitive oximetry and heart rate variability assessment, together with a urinary test for catecholamines in the morning for those patients with a high or low pretest probability for OSAS.

For those patients with intermediate probability, or those in whom other forms of SDB are sought, a more complete PSG will be available. This diagnostic test will be wireless, and capable of measuring a greater variety of physiological variables (e.g. blood pressure, arousal, brain activity). Static charged beds, sufficiently sensitive to measured respiration, heart rate and body movements, may solve this problem. They are currently available and under investigation. The accurate measurement of sound (amplitude, frequency, tone, pitch) will improve and possibly assist clinicians to determine the site of obstruction.

The current standard technique of sleep staging is based on a system developed in the 1960s for dealing with normal, healthy patients. This staging process is likely to change so that more subtle alterations in brain wave activity in response to drugs or diseased states can be identified. This may come in the form of power spectral analysis of the EEG waveform. Perhaps one day an accurate blood, urine or salivary test for sleepiness will be developed.

Standardized monitors of driving performance will be developed and may comprise computer-operated systems for use within the clinician's office. Since OSAS is prevalent and a risk to motorists, standardized assessments of sleepiness and driving skill may become part of the normal licensing procedure. New methods of assessing sleepiness while patients are at the wheel of their car (e.g. blink assessment, movement sensor in the steering wheel) will also be developed.

Primary care clinicians will probably assume responsibility for the diagnosis and management of most straightforward cases of OSAS, much as they do for most prevalent conditions, such as hypertension and asthma. However, cardiologists will become increasingly involved in the diagnosis and management of these patients, because OSAS causes and exacerbates cardiovascular disease. This focus on the part of cardiologists will be accompanied by diagnostic and management approaches centered on cardiovascular physiology, such as heart rate variability and nocturnal sympathetic tone.

Management

For the foreseeable future, the management of OSAS will remain centered around various forms of positive air pressure. The past decade has seen a flood of automated CPAP devices. With such a rapid rate of development, clinical trials cannot be completed before the next wave of devices becomes available. As a result, it is necessary to rely on a small number of clinical trials that are generic for a particular device. Given the patents covering the algorithms used by these automated positive-pressure airway devices, devices cannot and should not be assumed to be equal.

Just as positive inotropes have a very limited role in heart failure, drugs designed to increase the activity of the failing upper airway muscles are a long way off. Agents that prevent collapse by altering surface tension may be available in the future as inhalers or puffers similar to those used to treat asthma.

Upper airway muscle pacemakers have been studied, but unfortunately they usually awaken the patient with each impulse. Moreover, it is unclear which muscle needs to be stimulated and when in relation to the respiratory cycle. It is possible and likely, however, that new techniques will be developed that allow pacemakers to play a role in the management of OSAS.

A wider range of clinicians will be required to manage OSAS. In many countries, this work is currently limited to accredited sleep physicians. In the future, it is likely that the management of OSAS will be initiated by primary care physicians, in a similar way as in asthma and diabetes. It will be those patients requiring more elaborate PSG (e.g. if they have a moderate pretest probability of OSAS), those who have complex disease (e.g. kyphoscoliosis or heart failure) and those having difficulty tolerating treatment who will require the help of accredited sleep physicians, most of whom will have a training background in respiratory medicine.

Useful websites

www.sleepaus.on.net
The Australasian Sleep Association represents clinicians, scientists and researchers in the broad area of sleep in Australia and New Zealand.

www.aasmnet.org
The American Academy of Sleep Medicine is a professional membership organization dedicated to the advancement of sleep medicine and research.

www.aptweb.org
The Association of Polysomnographic Technologists is an international society of professionals dedicated to improving the quality of sleep and wakefulness in all people.

www.sleeptechnologists.com
The Australasian Sleep Technologists Association website was developed to encourage communication among people working in the fields of sleep medicine and sleep research.

www.sleepfoundation.org
The US National Sleep Foundation is an independent non-profit organization dedicated to improving public health and safety by achieving understanding of sleep and sleep disorders, and by supporting education, sleep-related research and advocacy.

www.nhlbi.nih.gov/about/ncsdr/
The US National Center on Sleep Disorders Research of the National Institutes of Health coordinates government-supported sleep research, training and education to improve health.

www.sleepapnea.org
The American Sleep Apnea Association (ASAA) is dedicated to reducing injury, disability and death from sleep apnea through education, awareness and research. The ASAA also promotes voluntary support groups.

www.sleeping.org.uk
The British Sleep Society is a professional organization for medical, healthcare and scientific workers. It aims to improve public health by promoting education and research into sleep and its disorders.

www.belsleep.org
The Belgian Association for the Study of Sleep disseminates information on the field of sleep among healthcare professionals and organizes regular scientific meetings.

www.esrs.org
The European Sleep Research Society is an international scientific non-profit organization promoting all aspects of sleep research. These include the publication of the *Journal of Sleep Research*, the organization of scientific meetings, the promotion of training and education, the dissemination of information and the establishment of fellowships and awards.

www.isat.ie
The Irish Sleep Apnoea Trust is a patient support group for sufferers and their families. It promotes awareness, understanding and treatment of sleep apnea through education, research and fundraising.

www.apss.org
The Associated Professional Sleep Societies (APSS) is a joint venture of the American Academy of Sleep Medicine and the Sleep Research Society.

www.1sleep.com
The International Sleep Medicine Association aims to be a complete source for sleep information and communication for all people interested in sleep and sleep disorders, and to improve sleep health by educating healthcare providers and the public.

Index

Useful websites

www.sleepaus.on.net
The Australasian Sleep Association represents clinicians, scientists and researchers in the broad area of sleep in Australia and New Zealand.

www.aasmnet.org
The American Academy of Sleep Medicine is a professional membership organization dedicated to the advancement of sleep medicine and research.

www.aptweb.org
The Association of Polysomnographic Technologists is an international society of professionals dedicated to improving the quality of sleep and wakefulness in all people.

www.sleeptechnologists.com
The Australasian Sleep Technologists Association website was developed to encourage communication among people working in the fields of sleep medicine and sleep research.

www.sleepfoundation.org
The US National Sleep Foundation is an independent non-profit organization dedicated to improving public health and safety by achieving understanding of sleep and sleep disorders, and by supporting education, sleep-related research and advocacy.

www.nhlbi.nih.gov/about/ncsdr/
The US National Center on Sleep Disorders Research of the National Institutes of Health coordinates government-supported sleep research, training and education to improve health.

www.sleepapnea.org
The American Sleep Apnea Association (ASAA) is dedicated to reducing injury, disability and death from sleep apnea through education, awareness and research. The ASAA also promotes voluntary support groups.

www.sleeping.org.uk
The British Sleep Society is a professional organization for medical, healthcare and scientific workers. It aims to improve public health by promoting education and research into sleep and its disorders.

www.belsleep.org
The Belgian Association for the Study of Sleep disseminates information on the field of sleep among healthcare professionals and organizes regular scientific meetings.

www.esrs.org
The European Sleep Research Society is an international scientific non-profit organization promoting all aspects of sleep research. These include the publication of the *Journal of Sleep Research*, the organization of scientific meetings, the promotion of training and education, the dissemination of information and the establishment of fellowships and awards.

www.isat.ie
The Irish Sleep Apnoea Trust is a patient support group for sufferers and their families. It promotes awareness, understanding and treatment of sleep apnea through education, research and fundraising.

www.apss.org
The Associated Professional Sleep Societies (APSS) is a joint venture of the American Academy of Sleep Medicine and the Sleep Research Society.

www.1sleep.com
The International Sleep Medicine Association aims to be a complete source for sleep information and communication for all people interested in sleep and sleep disorders, and to improve sleep health by educating healthcare providers and the public.

Index